Contents

INTRODUCTION

One of the most misunderstood mental health conditions is Borderline Personality Disorder (BPD). If you are like most people, you probably think that medication is the only way to treat this psychiatric illness. But there are many natural solutions that can help. Before going into these strategies, let's take a closer look at this often debilitating condition.

The sufferers of Borderline Personality Disorder (BPD) are well aware of the dark side of living with this disorder. To have BPD is to be confronted daily and without release through the years to an unstable mood, unregulated emotions, and a fear of rejection- as well as a whole lot of other symptoms that can make life unbearable.

Borderline personality disorder (BPD) is a serious mental health condition in which those affected can experience patterns of turbulent emotional states and long-term emotional instability. The BPD definition also includes characteristics such as impulsive actions, chaotic relationships, fluctuations in mood, self-image and general functioning. 2 The BPD definition also describes the likelihood of co-occurring mental health conditions such as anxiety, depression, and mood and eating disorders. BPD may also include an inclination towards substance abuse, self-harm and suicidal thoughts and actions.2 BPD affects the day-to-day lives of those suffering from this mental health condition. It can impact routines such as work, family life, and social activities. BPD typically begins by young adulthood whereby symptoms are more severe and gradually get better with age.

Borderline Personality Disorder In Adolescent is a mental disorder classified by unstable moods, difficulties with interpersonal relationships, and volatile and impulsive behavior, and it is typically diagnosed in early adulthood. Researchers are not positive exactly what causes borderline personality disorder at this point, but early evidence points to a high likelihood of a combination of genetic and environmental factors being involved.

One randomized control trial comparing DBT-A to psychodynamic therapy and CBT found that DBT-A was associated with increased reductions in depressive symptoms, borderline symptoms, self-harming behaviors, and suicidal ideation over the other treatments.

If you have borderline personality disorder, don't get discouraged. Many people with this disorder get better over time with treatment and can learn to live satisfying lives. Borderline personality disorder affects how you feel about yourself, how you relate to others and how you behave.

BPD appears to be a neurodevelopmental disorder, influenced by the person's genetics and brain development and shaped by early environment, including attachment and traumatic experiences. Childhood trauma such as sexual, emotional, or physical abuse also may lead to the onset of borderline personality disorder. Unstable relationships are a main symptom of BPD , and children with traumatic backgrounds or unhealthy family relationships may be more prone to developing BPD later in life.

CHAPTER ONE

What is borderline personality disorder

Borderline personality disorder is an illness marked by an ongoing pattern of varying moods, self-image, and behavior. These symptoms often result in impulsive actions and problems in relationships with other people. A person with borderline personality disorder may experience episodes of anger, depression, and anxiety that may last from a few hours to days. Recognizable symptoms typically show up during adolescence (teenage years) or early adulthood, but early symptoms of the illness can occur during childhood.

What Causes Borderline Personality Disorder (BPD)?

Specific borderline personality disorder causes are unknown. This is partially because many mental health experts now feel that the term BPD is vague or misleading. Instead, BPD may include a wide range of causes unique to each individual who suffers from the condition.2 Some of the potential borderline personality disorder causes include genetic, family, social, neurological and environmental factors.1,2 Depending on the individual, there may be a number of risk factors involved in the development of BPD, such as;

- Childhood abandonment
- Unstable family life
- Lack of communication within the family
- Sexual, physical or emotional trauma and abuse
- A BPD diagnosis in another family member
- Potential structural or physical changes within the brain
- General impulsive or aggressive personality traits
- Being female, as more females are diagnosed with BPD
- Being predisposed to other psychiatric conditions

Symptoms

Borderline personality disorder affects how you feel about yourself, how you relate to others and how you behave.

Signs and symptoms may include:

- Impulsive and risky behavior, such as gambling, reckless driving, unsafe sex, spending sprees, binge eating or drug abuse, or sabotaging success by suddenly quitting a good job or ending a positive relationship
- Suicidal threats or behavior or self-injury, often in response to fear of separation or rejection
- Wide mood swings lasting from a few hours to a few days, which can include intense happiness, irritability, shame or anxiety
- Ongoing feelings of emptiness
- Inappropriate, intense anger, such as frequently losing your temper, being sarcastic or bitter, or having physical fights

- An intense fear of abandonment, even going to extreme measures to avoid real or imagined separation or rejection
- A pattern of unstable intense relationships, such as idealizing someone one moment and then suddenly believing the person doesn't care enough or is cruel
- Rapid changes in self-identity and self-image that include shifting goals and values, and seeing yourself as bad or as if you don't exist at all
- Periods of stress-related paranoia and loss of contact with reality, lasting from a few minutes to a few hours

Sufferers of BPD tend to do whatever they can to avoid any form of perceived abandonment or rejection, having extreme reactions to things such as a vacation or someone being a few minutes late to an appointment. These feelings can trigger intense anger and lead to impulsive and self-harming behavior. Sometimes these behaviors include suicidal tendencies, although usually, the intent is not to follow through. Relationships are tough for those who suffer from BPD as feelings can quickly shift from one of intense love to a feeling of the recipient not caring enough or not being there for them. Usually, BPD causes turmoil in all relationships, not just personal ones, but can extend into the workplace as well. Those who suffer from BPD are extremely sensitive to their environment, and seemingly innocuous events can be a trigger.

Impulsive thoughts and actions can lead to self-harming actions like substance abuse, reckless driving, eating disorders, self-mutilation, risky sexual behavior, and inappropriate spending. According to Psychiatric Times, 50 to 70 percent of individuals diagnosed with borderline personality disorder also suffer from a substance abuse disorder, usually involving alcohol abuse. An unstable sense of self, or self-image is indicative of BPD also. This can lead to quick changes in goals, careers and the like. Opinions of self tend to fluctuate from high to low rapidly. Sufferers of BPD sometimes describe "out-of-body" experiences and feelings of separateness.

Who Is Affected by Borderline Personality Disorder?

Borderline Personality Disorder is more common than you might think. It affects an estimated 1.4% of the U.S. population (over 4 million people), but it could be as high as 5.9% (over 19 million). Unlike ADD/ADHD and Autism Spectrum Disorder (ASD), which are typically identified in children and adolescents. BPD often begins in a person's late teens or early 20s. BPD is more commonly seen in women, who make up 75% of those diagnosed with the condition. However, the high prevalence in women may be due in part to the fact that many men with BPD are misdiagnosed with depression or post-traumatic stress disorder (PTSD). BPD is also often misdiagnosed as bipolar disorder.

Borderline Personality Disorder or Bipolar Disorder?

BPD is often misdiagnosed as bipolar disorder. Though their symptoms can be similar (mood swings, impulsiveness, and outbursts), their diagnoses are completely different. Bipolar disorder is identified by alternating periods of depression and mania. Those periods can last from a few days to several months.

By contrast, borderline personality disorder is distinguished by a long-term pattern of frequently shifting moods and behaviors. These episodes are typically triggered by interactions with other people. People with BPD are more likely to have other mental health issues as well as some type of childhood trauma.

Complications

Borderline personality disorder can damage many areas of your life. It can negatively affect intimate relationships, jobs, school, social activities and self-image, resulting in:

- Conflict-filled relationships, marital stress or divorce
- Self-injury, such as cutting or burning, and frequent hospitalizations
- Involvement in abusive relationships

- Repeated job changes or losses
- Not completing an education
- Multiple legal issues, such as jail time
- Unplanned pregnancies, sexually transmitted infections, motor vehicle accidents and physical fights due to impulsive and risky behavior
- Attempted or completed suicide

In addition, you may have other mental health disorders, such as:

- Bipolar disorder
- Post-traumatic stress disorder (PTSD)
- Attention-deficit/hyperactivity disorder (ADHD)
- Depression
- Alcohol or other substance misuse
- Anxiety disorders
- Eating disorders
- Other personality disorders

How do I know if I have borderline personality disorder?

A licensed mental health professional such as a psychiatrist, psychologist, or clinical social worker experienced in diagnosing and treating mental disorders can diagnose borderline personality disorder, based on a thorough interview and a discussion about symptoms. A careful and thorough medical exam can also help rule out other possible causes of symptoms.

The mental health professional may ask about symptoms and personal and family medical histories, including any history of mental illness. This information can help determine the best treatment.

4 Types of Borderline Personality Disorder

Discouraged

People with this subtype resemble the core BPD subtype identified by researchers. In fact, people who suffer from the discouraged subtype tend to be clingy, co-dependent, and less assertive. Also, they're often compliant and agreeable in a variety of situations.

However, they're likely to feel depressed, powerless, and may even struggle with their anger. Thus, individuals with this subtype are susceptible to self-harm and suicidal thoughts or actions.

Self-Destructive

People with self-destructive traits tend to be self-loathing, involved in risky behavior, and are usually introverted. These individuals cast an unusual pattern of conforming to other people's beliefs and expectations then acting out in anger.

Such anger and frustration may not only be directed to others but also towards the individuals themselves. In fact, people with self-destructive traits tend to have an increased rate of suicide. Also, they're known to share characteristics of depression disorders.

Impulsive

People who exhibit the borderline impulsive subtype are usually characterized as attention-seeking and risk-taking. People describe these individuals as seductive and even charismatic.

However, they're susceptible to self-harming behaviors and suicidal thoughts and actions. Many people with borderline impulsive disorder share similar traits with other personality disorders. For instance, they can be overly dramatic, emotional, and even at times unpredictable.

Petulant

People who have petulant borderline disorder are often critical, pessimistic, and easily disappointed. They may feel offended and decide to react out of rage or anger. Feeling unwanted, unloved, or unworthy are all big trigger points for these individuals.

In fact, these individuals are often erratic in relationships and demonstrate the "push-pull" philosophy. Meaning that they usually feel a strong or deep bond with a person, and they begin to push them away. These individuals also exhibit symptoms of paranoid personality disorder and even some traits of depression disorders.

5 Tips for Borderline Personality Disorder Family Members

If you are struggling with how to handle a family member with BPD, here are some practical strategies that can help:

1. Don't Tiptoe

Though it might feel like a natural response to the radical, emotional swings of BPD, don't tiptoe around the person for fear of setting them off. Hiding your thoughts and feelings to avoid a confrontation isn't healthy.

2. Avoid Isolating

Feelings of hopelessness can lead to isolation. Force yourself to stay connected with your lifelines: family and friends. Frequent conversations with safe and trusted people can provide you with support, understanding, and encouragement.

3. Focus on Emotions, Not Words

It's easy to react to the angry words a BPD person is saying, but condition yourself to remain calm and focus on the emotions behind their statements. People with BPD need acknowledgment of their pain, not lengthy explanations regarding the appropriateness of their words.

4. Learn the 3 C's

It's normal to feel responsible for the frequent ups and downs that a BPD patient experiences. Learn to let yourself off the hook with these 3 C's:

- I didn't cause it.
- I can't cure it.
- 3. I can't control it.

5. Go Slow

Recovery is a process. It's a marathon, not a sprint, so pace yourself. Set realistic goals and expect occasional setbacks. Taking baby steps will give someone with BPD a greater chance at succeeding in the long run.

What Are the Treatment Options?

There are three common treatment options for BPD: talk therapy, medication, and day treatment. Talk therapy centers on the thoughts that can cause certain behaviors and actions. With this therapy, people learn how to control distress and learn how to cope with intense emotions.

While there are no current medications that treat BPD, certain medications can decrease the underlying symptoms. For instance, a doctor may request antidepressants, mood stabilizers, or even antipsychotics for a patient to take. Keep in mind that usually, talk therapy and medication are used in combination with one another. That way, a patient can talk through their emotions while reducing their symptoms. However, day treatment provides a more intensive treatment plan. This treatment is usually for emergency purposes. It's for those who may be headed towards a crisis. With day treatment, a patient will experience accelerated therapy and perhaps even alternative medications to prevent a crisis from occurring.

Borderline personality disorder has historically been viewed as difficult to treat. But with newer, evidence-based treatment, many people with borderline personality disorder experience fewer and less severe symptoms, improved functioning, and an improved quality of life. It is important for patients with borderline personality disorder to receive evidence-based, specialized treatment from an appropriately-trained mental health professional. Other types of treatment, or treatment provided by a provider who is not appropriately trained, may not benefit the patient.

Many factors affect the length of time it takes for symptoms to improve once treatment begins, so it is important for people with borderline personality disorder and their loved ones to be patient and to receive appropriate support during treatment.

It is important to seek and stick with treatment.

NIMH-funded studies indicate that borderline personality disorder patients who don't receive adequate treatment are more likely to develop other chronic medical or mental illnesses and are less likely to make healthy lifestyle choices. Borderline personality disorder is also associated with a significantly higher rate of self-harm and suicidal behavior than the general population.

What Is Borderline Personality Disorder In Adolescent?

Borderline personality disorder (BPD) in adolescents is defined as a 1-year pattern of immature personality development with disturbances in at least five of the following domains: efforts to avoid abandonment, unstable interpersonal relationships, identity disturbance, impulsivity, suicidal and self-mutilating behaviors, affective instability, chronic feelings of emptiness, inappropriate intense anger, and stress-related paranoid ideation. BPD can be reliably diagnosed in adolescents as young as 11 years. The available epidemiological studies suggest that the prevalence of BPD in the general population of adolescents is around 3%. The clinical prevalence of BPD ranges from 11% in adolescents consulting at an outpatient clinic to 78% in suicidal adolescents attending an emergency department.

What causes borderline personality disorder in teens?

For example, childhood abuse and neglect, as well as parental separation or loss, have been linked to borderline personality in adults and teens. Research has also found that kids whose parents have serious mental health conditions (e.g., depression, substance abuse or antisocial personality) are also at greater risk for BPD.

Symptoms of Borderline Personality Disorder In Adolescent

- Self-harm

- Depression
- Fear of abandonment or rejection
- Difficulty maintaining relationships
- Frequent and intense changes in mood
- Impulsive and risky behavior
- Paranoia

Symptoms, such as instability in interpersonal relationships, impulsive behavior, chronic emptiness, and unstable sense of self, may look different in teens. It may also sometimes be difficult to distinguish between symptoms of BPD and normal teenage challenges.

Diagnosis

On consultation, many adolescents (particularly those in an emergency or crisis situation) present with BPTs. When faced with a heterogeneous, unstable clinical profile, the challenge for the clinician is to detect the BPTs' persistence over time, interactions during the individual and family interviews, and what is reported by the adolescent about the relationships with his/her peers at school, on social networks, and, potentially, in hospital. The diagnostic challenge is to detect the "duration" criterion (1year for DSM-V6) and recurrent, abnormal functioning in several affective contexts. Another common presentation is nonsuicidal self-injury (NSSI). In recent studies, 58% of suicidal BPD adolescents reported NSSI, whereas 51.7% of female adolescents engaging in NSSI met criteria for BPD. Suicidal and NSSI behaviors should always prompt the clinician to screen for BPD. For the adolescent's physician, the syndrome might also manifest itself as repeated somatic problems or as poor adherence to the treatment of somatic complaint. Even though a growing number of clinicians recognize the clinical existence of BPD in the adolescent, there is still much debate as to the most appropriate way of conceptualizing this disorder (ie, in categorical or dimensional terms) as a single-factor or multifactor entity. In routine clinical practice, many clinicians adopt a categorical approach and refer to the diagnostic categories given in international classifications, including the DSM-V.6 However, several researchers have argued for an integrated developmental approach that takes account of both normal personality development and its anomalies. The clinician can therefore choose categorical or dimensional approaches for the diagnosis of BPD, together with a psychopathological approach for the identification of a BPO.

What are the challenges in making the diagnosis?

The current diagnostic criteria for borderline personality disorder allow for 256 different combinations of symptoms that could lead to a diagnosis. Clinicians thus may find it challenging to make a diagnosis of borderline personality disorder. Because of their limited time to spend with patients, clinicians can look for several key factors to help them decide whether further assessment for the disorder is necessary.

The most important factor is whether the difficulties have been long standing or, for adolescents, present for at least 1 year. If there is a sudden change in functioning or new symptoms, a diagnosis of borderline personality disorder is less likely according to the DSM-IV-TR definition. Having difficulties in multiple areas is another important factor. For example, suicidality or self-harm without problems with mood or relationships is less likely to be borderline personality disorder, whereas a history of suicide attempts along with impulsive substance use and problems with chronic feelings of emptiness and anger is more suggestive of a diagnosis.

If the diagnosis of borderline personality disorder is not made, an affected person may end up with several diagnoses of comorbid disorders, none of which responds to common treatments. For example, patients who have major depressive disorder and comorbid borderline personality disorder generally do not respond as well to antidepressant medications as patients do who have major depressive disorder alone.

Prognosis

For adults with BPD, the symptoms of the condition typically gradually decline with age, particularly past the age of 40. The progression and outlook for teens with the condition are less clear, although appropriate treatment can significantly improve the management of symptoms.

According to a review published in 2015, the remission rate for adolescents could range from 50% to 65%, however, it's also possible that some symptoms could remain even though some teens no longer met the diagnostic criteria for BPD.

How should patients be informed of their diagnosis?

Once a diagnosis of borderline personality disorder has been established, it is important to inform the patient of the diagnosis and discuss the implications for treatment options and outcomes. There is no evidence to indicate that informing patients of the diagnosis causes problems, so it is unfortunate that this important step is often omitted. When informing a patient about a suspected diagnosis of borderline personality disorder, clinical experience suggests that it is helpful to show the patient the list of diagnostic criteria and explain why the diagnosis is being considered. Educating patients about the increasing number of specific treatments and the good prognosis with gradually resolving symptoms can also help reduce their anxiety about a diagnosis that is highly stigmatized in the medical system and the general population. Even a single psychoeducation session could help to reduce symptoms, as was found in a randomized trial in which 30 of 50 late adolescent women found to have borderline personality disorder were randomly assigned to attend such a session within a week after being told about their diagnosis.

Risk Factors For Borderline Personality Disorder In Adolescent

The risk factors for borderline personality in adolescents are very similar to the risk factors in adults. In fact, many of the environmental risk factors for BPD occur during childhood. Some of the factors that may increase the risk of BPD include:

Family history

Research has also found that kids whose parents have serious mental health conditions (such as depression, substance abuse, or antisocial personality) are also at greater risk for BPD.

Brain differences

Research has also found that people who have BPD often have changes in areas of the brain that are associated with the regulation of emotions and impulses.

Genetic influences

In addition, there are likely biological risk factors for BPD, such as a genetic component of the disorder that is inherited.

Environmental factors

Childhood abuse and neglect, as well as parental separation or loss, have been linked to borderline personality in adults and teens.

Is Borderline Personality Disorder Hereditary?

Those suffering from borderline personality disorder may have certain regions of the brain affected also. According to NHS, MRIs done on people with BPD indicate that their prefrontal cortex, which helps to regulate emotions, self-control, and behavior, may be smaller than normal or not as developed. Conversely, the amygdala seems to be overactive in those suffering from BPD, which leads to heightened emotions and more intense emotional reactions. Neurotransmitters, chemicals messengers in the brain responsible for the regulation of sleep, learning, and mood, may also be at lower levels in those diagnosed with BPD. While certain personality traits indicative of borderline personality disorder like impulsivity and aggression may be inherited, brain formation and development are not entirely genetic; they are affected by environmental factors as well.

Prevention

If you are worried that your adolescent may be at risk for developing BPD based on either environmental risk factors (e.g., trauma exposure) or biological risk factors (e.g., a first-degree relative with the disorder), some experts believe that there are ways to modify the course of the condition. Kids who experience externalizing disorders such as oppositional defiant disorder (ODD) and attention-deficit hyperactivity disorder (ADHD) appear to be more likely to develop BPD symptoms in adolescence.The presence of depression in adolescence appears to predict BPD during adulthood. This suggests that early detection and the use of specific therapeutic interventions to address those symptoms may be helpful in changing the course of the disorder.

Management

Before initiating treatment, the therapist should obtain informed consent from both the youngster and his/her parent(s), in order to comply with the legislation and pave the way to a positive therapeutic alliance between the youngster, the parent(s), and the healthcare professionals. As with any therapeutic intervention in adolescent medicine, parental involvement is critical. Considering the long duration of BPD and the unpredictability of its management, it is preferable to take the time to build a solid alliance with the youngster and his/her family, based on the provision of clear information about the pathology and its treatment, an evaluation of the adolescent's level of commitment, and the establishment of realistic treatment objectives. Family interviews are thus an essential component of any therapeutic intervention. Integrated care programs that offer an opportunity to review therapeutic transactions as a team and to re-evaluate the treatment options from time to time are more effective than a therapeutic intervention by an individual therapist. Regardless of the patient's status (ie, an outpatient or a partial or full inpatient), he/she must receive continuous, specialist care, with the management organized around outpatient consultations.

Living With Borderline Personality Disorder

Living with borderline personality disorder (BPD) poses some challenges. Intense emotional pain and feelings of emptiness, desperation, anger, hopelessness, and loneliness are common. These symptoms can affect every part of your life. Despite the challenges, many people with BPD learn how to cope with the symptoms so they can live fulfilling lives.

Your Physical Health and BPD

Unfortunately, BPD can also have a major impact on your physical health. BPD is associated with a variety of conditions, including chronic pain disorders such as fibromyalgia and chronic fatigue syndrome, arthritis, obesity, diabetes, and other serious health problems. BPD is also associated with less-than-healthy lifestyle choices such as smoking, alcohol use, and lack of regular exercise.

Your Relationships and BPD

BPD can have a major impact on your relationships. In fact, having difficulties in relationships is one of the primary symptoms of BPD. People with BPD can have many arguments and conflicts with loved ones or a lot of relationships that repeatedly break up.

BPD and the Law

Some of the behaviors associated with BPD can lead to legal problems as well. The anger associated with it can lead to aggression (e.g., assaulting others, throwing objects, or acting out against others' personal property). Impulsive behaviors, such as driving recklessly, misusing substances, shoplifting, or engaging in other illegal acts, can also lead to trouble.

Coping With BPD Symptoms

People with BPD do not have to resign themselves to a life of emotional pain. There are a number of things you can do to help you cope with the symptoms.

Your Work and BPD

Work, school, or other productive pursuits can give us a sense of purpose in life. Unfortunately, BPD can interfere with your success at work or school. Since BPD has such an impact on relationships, people with BPD may find themselves in trouble with co-workers, bosses, teachers, or other authority figures. The intense emotional changes may also impact work or school; you may have to be absent more often due to emotional concerns or hospitalization.

Have a Safety Plan

BPD causes very painful emotions and, as a result, it is not uncommon for mental health emergencies (for example, active suicidality) to arise. For this reason, it is critical for you to have a safety plan in place before a crisis happens.

Discouraged Foods for Borderline Personality Disorder

Foods that are heavily processed can lead to fatigue and mood swings, which are never good for people with BPD. This also includes foods that have a significant amount of added sugar to them, such as sweetened drinks and desserts. Processed meats, refined grains, and low-quality dairy products are all foods that you should stay far away from when you are working to get over BPD.

Breakfast Diet for Borderline Personality Disorder

Breakfast is often revered as the most important meal of the day, and with that being said, it is important to choose foods that will help you cope with the symptoms of BPD for your breakfast meal. Foods that are rich in magnesium have been shown to drastically improve brain health. Foods with whole grains, such as whole-wheat bread, would be an excellent addition to your breakfast. Adding just a slice of toasted whole wheat bread, or whole wheat cereals, and a handful of nuts, (specifically peanuts, almonds, and cashews), and a dash of dark chocolate, is a delicious, healthy breakfast that not only supports the health of your body, but the health of your mind as well.

Lunch Diet for Borderline Personality Disorder

To prepare the best lunch suited for someone with BPD, you will want to get some walnuts and some cold water fish, such as salmon, and add some plants such as avocado, cauliflower, or spinach leaves to the mix to create a balanced lunch that has both fatty acids and additional magnesium. If you choose to live a vegan or vegetarian lifestyle, then you can substitute the cold water fish with some tofu for a more magnesium-rich diet.

Dinner Diet for Borderline Personality Disorder

Dinner is usually the time of day that requires the heartiest of meals. For this large meal, you are going to want to look toward quinoa, black beans, and edamame (soybeans that are still in the pod), which are all rich in magnesium, as well as grass-fed beef, brussels sprouts, and cold water fish for your increased fatty acid intake. There are many combinations of meals to make with these foods, and finding the perfect mix will be part of your journey to living life coping with BPD.

Drinks for Borderline Personality Disorder

There are also a variety of drinks that you can make to improve your ability to handle BPD as well. As Vitamin C is important, orange juice would be a lovely addition to your life. A dark chocolate smoothie would also be a soothing treat for summer days, while also increasing your magnesium intake. Adding strawberries can both increase your Vitamin C and add some flavor to your smoothie as well. Flax seed oil and hemp oil are both sources of fatty acids, although it can alter the taste of your drink a little bit, so be prepared for that. Milk is an excellent source of Vitamin D, which is something that people with BPD should look for.

Fruits for Borderline Personality Disorder

The most common fruit is, of course, going to be oranges. Any citrus fruit will do well though, so you can add lemons, limes, and grapefruits to your fruit intake as well. Strawberries are also high in Vitamin C, making them a wonderful addition to any diet. Tomatoes, which are scientifically considered a fruit, are also high in

Vitamin C, making them a wonderful way to spruce up dinners and lunches.

Natural Remedies and Herbs for Borderline Personality Disorder (BPD)

There are natural borderline personality disorder treatments available which include:

- Kava Kava - A borderline personality disorder treatment like kava kava can help to reduce anxiety and calm down intense emotional states.
- Valerian - Valerian can help to control anxiety and depression and help people with BPD fight intense urges.
- St. John’s Wort - St. John's Wort is one of the most effective BPD natural remedies because it has natural mood enhancing properties which can support those who are facing depression and anxiety.
- Omega-3 Fatty Acids - Omega-3 fatty acids are shown to help reduce aggression, depression and other BPD symptoms.

- Yokukansan - BPD natural remedies also include the Japanese herbal treatment, yokukansan which helps suppress feelings of agitation and mood swings.
- Yerbamate - Yerbamate is a natural anti-anxiety herb which helps to stabilize mood and reduce BPD symptoms.

CHAPTER TWO

Strategies for Parenting a Teen, Child with Borderline Personality Disorder

Parenting BPD teenagers and children requires specific skills. They can't and won't respond well to the way you parent your non-BPD kids. The following approaches have been successful for many parents struggling to raise someone with this personality disorder.

Set Boundaries

Whether they like it or not, your child must live within boundaries and limits. Work with your child to create limits (one at a time) that work for everyone, and explain that they're in place for love and security. Create your boundaries based on what your family needs, but one that is important for all families dealing with BPD is a zero-tolerance policy for violence, abuse, and destruction (all part of BPD). Establish simple consequences that you can enforce consistently.

Clear Communication

Someone with BPD can misinterpret messages, read into expressions, and internalize conversations in negative ways. They also easily feel humiliated and react strongly at what you intended to be an innocent comment. When talking with your child, use simple, straightforward, clear communication. Leave nothing open for interpretation. Be mindful of your nonverbal communication and tone of voice, too; for example, adopt a neutral, relaxed posture and even tone.

Validate

To reassure them and calm the storm when it rages, validate them. Listen fully, reflect their words and feelings back to them so they feel heard. Reassure them that their feelings are legitimate, and help them express their emotions verbally.

Lower your expectations and adjust goals

While this is the opposite of parenting non-BPD children, it's essential for your child or teen with the disorder. Keep expectations simple and few.

Help them set realistic goals and very small steps to achieve them. Otherwise, you'll risk an overwhelmed, angry outburst driven by their belief that you're trying to get rid of them.

Create Calm

BPD is dominated by chaos, for your child, you, and the rest of the family. To counter this, create a home environment that is calm and inviting. Make a comfortable space for destressing, breathing, meditating, and stretching. Everyone in your family can benefit from a secure deescalating zone.

Handling Conflict

It can seem like conflict is constant, so wanting to avoid it makes sense. It does not make sense to your child, and they'll let you know it. Address problems calmly, quietly, and non-judgmentally.

Treatments

While BPD is a serious and complex condition, there are effective treatments available that can help manage and reduce symptoms. Getting an accurate diagnosis and the use of appropriate treatments is important.

Psychotherapy

Several types of psychotherapy including cognitive-behavioral therapy (CBT) and dialectical behavior therapy (DBT) may be effective with teens with borderline personality.

- CBT can be useful for helping people learn to recognize and change negative thoughts that contribute to symptoms of the condition.
- DBT helps people address destructive behaviors, learn new skills, and find ways of tolerating distress and difficult emotions.

DBT has also been adapted for use specifically with adolescents. Dialectical-behavioral therapy for adolescents (DBT-A) involves individual psychotherapy and family skills training.

Medications

- Anti-anxiety medications may also be prescribed on a short-term basis to help manage some symptoms, however, benzodiazepines should never be prescribed to treat BPD.

- Melatonin may also be useful for treating insomnia, which is often present with BPD.
- Research suggests that second-generation antipsychotics can be useful for managing suicide risk when used in conjunction with psychotherapy.
- Medications such as Ritalin (methylphenidate) and selective serotonin reuptake inhibitors (SSRIs) may also be prescribed to treat co-occurring ADHD and depression.
-

Tips for Dealing with Borderline Personality Disorder

It can be confusing to decide which way to go when you have an intense emotion. It would be even harder to control your emotions when you have borderline personality disorder (BPD). The most common symptoms of BPD are self-harming behaviors, erratic mood shifts, intense emotional experiences, suicidal thoughts, and problems with impulsive behaviors.All these issues are related to emotion dysregulation, which is the reason why you are going to have strong emotional responses to different events. Dealing with borderline personality disorder is never easy, but you can take steps to make things more manageable.

Practice Mindfulness

The idea is to experience the emotion without trying to block it. Be mindful about what you are feeling. Do not suppress your emotion; instead, accept it for what it is and learn to move on.

Keep Yourself Busy

One of the most important skills to develop when dealing with borderline personality disorder is to keep yourself busy. Do not surrender to the emotion you are having. Instead, go for a highly engaging activity, such as dancing, walking, or something that distracts you from how you are feeling now. Keep in mind that watching TV or spending time on computer is never engaging enough. Look for something else.

Practice Deep Breathing

Controlling your breathing pattern will always help make things easier. Deep breathing relaxes your mind and helps you stay in control of things, making it one of the best tips for dealing with borderline personality disorder. Find a quiet place and take slow, deep breaths. Focus only on your breathing and feel your stomach rising and falling while you breathe. You can also try other relaxation exercises, such as progressive muscle relaxation.

Enjoy Some Music

You can use music sensibly to change your emotions. You have to select what may help create an emotion that is complete opposite of how you are feeling at a particular time. It means that if you are feeling sad, you may play upbeat music. In case you are feeling anxious, try listening to slow, relaxing music to feel better.

Do Not React Quickly

You need to develop a habit of taking some time before reacting to any situation. In most cases, those self-harming thoughts would pass in a few minutes. It means that you need to wait until the peak of those strong emotional reactions is passed. Simply get an egg timer from the kitchen and set it for 15 minutes. This will help you ride out the emotion.

Take a Warm Bath

When you are not feeling great and emotionally very week, a good way to relax your body is to take a warm bath. The sensations of the warm water will help divert your attention and relax your muscles as well. Using some essential oils would also help make your baths even more relaxing and beneficial.

Stay Grounded All the Time

Do not let your current emotion put you in a position where your previous emotions also start affecting your mind and take better of you. Stay grounded to avoid feeling 'zoned out', and you can do it by doing simple things like grabbing an ice cube in your hand. Sometimes, snapping a rubber band against your hand would also help you get out of the vicious circle of negative thoughts.

Use the Help of a Therapist

Even after trying certain things, you may still have to work with a therapist who explains the best ways of dealing with borderline personality disorder. Your therapist would use different therapies to make it easier for you to control your emotions.

- A popular option is Dialectical Behavior Therapy (DBT), which has a good success record and helps you learn how to regulate your emotions. The therapy also teaches you mindfulness skills and explains how to develop frustration tolerance, identify your emotions, and strengthen your psychosocial skills.
- Schema-Focused therapy is another option your therapist may use. This treatment approach is actually a mix of cognitive behavioral therapy and other therapy approaches. The therapy helps restructure your perceptions to help you have a stable self-image. Your therapist will work with

you directly to help produce desired results.

While there are therapies and techniques available to help you with your disorder, you need to describe your emotions in full detail to help your therapist determine the best treatment approach for you.

For this, you will have to learn about your emotions and know how to identify your physical and emotional feelings. It is not enough to tell your therapist that you feel a sinking in the pit of your stomach when you are dealing with certain situations, but you should be able to pinpoint exactly what triggers that feeling. This feeling could be related to anxiety or nervousness, and if you know that, it would be easier to bring things under control.

Another important thing is to work with your therapist and learn how you make and follow a set schedule. You are less likely to feel stressed when you schedule for things like sleep and meal times. Sleep deprivation and fluctuations in blood sugar levels can directly affect your emotional wellbeing.

Pray

Are you a religious or spiritual person? If you are or have considered attending religious ceremonies, praying and attending weekly congregations can be tremendously helpful in times of extreme stress.

Help Someone Else

Do something nice for someone else. It doesn't have to be something big; you can walk to the nearest store, buy a pack of gum and give the cashier a smile and say "have a great day." It may sound silly, but small gestures like this can really reduce emotional pain and connect you to the outside world.

Things Not To Do With Someone With Borderline Personality

Do you know the things you should do or the things you should say to someone with borderline personality disorder (BPD)? If not, join the millions of family, friends, and/or coworkers who don't. It is challenging to know exactly what to say, how to say it, and when to say it to avoid problems, challenges, or conflicts. Things can get worse if there are other individuals in the environment with an undiagnosed BPD.Despite these truths, compassion and understanding is the best tool to use.

Learning how to support someone diagnosed with BPD will require the acknowledgment that boundaries need to remain firm. Setting boundaries create a set of rules that can help confrontations or arguments dissolve more quickly. To begin setting these boundaries it is important not to:

Feel emotionally destroyed by impulsive remarks or behaviors:

Some individuals with BPD struggle with anger management and impulsivity. The foundation of relational problems is often anger and impulsivity. If you are feeling devalued or completely disrespected, make that known to the person and then create boundaries that make it clear you will not tolerate any abuse. If this does not help, gradually distance yourself until boundaries are "reset."

Allow boundary crossings:

Some individuals require you to maintain strong boundaries at all times. No questions asked. No doubt about it. You can't allow them to push boundaries with manipulation, seduction, or control.

Engage in codependent behaviors:

Co-dependence describes two individuals who lose their own identities, values, belief systems, feelings, thoughts, etc. due to an unhealthy fusion of two individuals in a relationship. Co-dependency may come across to others as "sweet," "romantic," or even "charming" until the truth comes out. In families, co-dependency can come across as "closeness" or "supportive." When co-dependence develops, the individual with BPD may control and manipulate or feel vulnerable if the relationship does not work out. If you begin to feel "suffocated" or responsible for how they ultimately feel, clarify the boundaries of the relationship and then empathize with them. Some individuals with BPD struggle with feelings of abandonment and will do almost anything to decrease these feelings.

Normalize things and minimize your intuition:

If it appears that something is truly wrong, something is most likely wrong. Everyone gets angry. Everyone experiences intense emotions. And everyone will over-react at some point in their lives. But if these behaviors are intense and repeated, attention should be paid to the behavior. Minimizing it or reducing its significance won't help anything. We aren't being helpful by minimizing.

Be pulled in by unsubstantiated fears of abandonment:

I once counseled a young lady who exhibited every single symptom of BPD but was way too young to be diagnosed at the time. When she became a teenager she started dating a lot of guys. In almost every relationship, she ended up losing the guy because she pushed them away with her desperate attempts to avoid the anxiety and negative thought patterns that would arise every time the guy would temporarily leave her. Most individuals with BPD have an intolerance of aloneness, loneliness, or being alone. This can result in unhealthy patterns of behaviors. You want to be careful with reinforcing these fears by how you respond. You can comfort the person or reassure them without enabling.

Be manipulated by cyclical chaos:

Chaos that occurs in cycles such as every spring, every school year, every anniversary, or every holiday may be intentional or unintentional behavior. In any case, you will want to avoid getting pulled into the person's cycle. If the cycle is manipulative and intentional, you really don't want to allow the person to gain that much control over you or anyone else. Disrupt the cycle by deterring it, blocking it, or switching up your plans. If cycles are unintentional, a more therapeutic approach should be utilized. You can't truly help the person if you get pulled in emotionally.

Be the "go to" person at ALL times:

Being the "go to" person is something that makes most of us feel loved, needed, and respected. But for some individuals with BPD, becoming the "go to" person may also mean that you will become the one most manipulated and controlled. The individual may begin to believe that they are "so very close to you" and "in your good graces" that you will always go the extra mile. Again, it's great to be needed but with boundaries.

Become emotional "prey":

In some relationships with individuals with BPD, you can easily feel like you are "prey." I once had a client tell me they felt their son would "use me for money and then discard me when he got ready." Individuals who are not in treatment for BPD and who may have sociopathic traits lack empathy. Keep boundaries, make your needs known, and create space between you and the other person as needed.

Feed into a need for attention/validation:

Not all individuals with BPD seek attention or validation from others. But some do.

Triangulation (i.e., bringing 3 or more people into an argument) is often a "vehicle" used to either obtain validation from someone else or get attention. Most people seek validation from people they trust and this is healthy. But some individuals seek validation to feel supported in doing things that aren't okay. For example, someone with BPD may misperceive the intentions of a loved one and believe that they are being "treated like a child." This individual may go to a close family member to gossip which causes this person to want to get involved in the argument and "make things better." To avoid feeding into this behavior, minimizing over-exaggerations or harmful gossiping can be helpful.

Always go the extra mile:

Going the extra mile is a wonderful thing to do. It's something we all hope someone will do for us. However, boundaries need to remain firm as needed and respected by the individual who chooses to manipulate the relationship.

Get pulled into the drama triangle:

Triangulation is a term used to describe an individual who often gets more than 2 people involved in a chaotic situation which results in more chaos. Instead of solving the problem with the person the problem started with, the individual may gossip to others who then feel compelled to intervene. But this intervention only makes things worse. To avoid this kind of triangulation, you can avoid discussing the incident with others who have nothing to do with the initial problem.

Look affected by attempts to control, manipulate, or dominate:

Any sign of emotional distress, agitation, anger, or even pleasure can give way too much information away to someone who intends to manipulate or control you. Some individuals are so keen to the emotions of others that they are able to decide how to "make their next move" in the relationship to remain in control. For example, I once counseled a young male with BPD who would report details of his life to me and then pause to see if I would respond in the fashion he had predicted. With this young man, I became almost stoic and would “downplay” some of his attempts to get a strong reaction from me. Sometimes having this response can change the entire encounter for the better.

Believe they are capable of “snapping out of it”:

Individuals diagnosed with BPD are not able to just “snap out of it.” They are being influenced by a variety of genetic, environmental, and social components that are also altered or influenced by personality, thought patterns, and/or learned behavior. “Snapping out of it” is not easy.

Get into a “routine” or habit:

Routines and habitual behavior can be helpful. But with some individuals with BPD, you don’t want to get into the habit of allowing certain things such as calls after hours, visits to your home without announcing it, borrowing your things and never returning them, driving your car and keeping it longer than they should, etc. Once you allow this kind of behavior to always occur, you will have a difficult time setting the boundary.

Normalize sexual promiscuity or risky behaviors:

Normalization of risky or inappropriate behaviors will only make things worse. Some individuals with BPD tend to push limits, engage in risky behaviors, or seek stimulation in ways that are unhealthy. For example, a male with BPD may engage in frequent binge drinking of alcohol and have multiple unsafe intimate relationships with others while being married and holding a great position at a law firm. This pattern of behavior may continue if others begin to normalize the behavior in an effort to make him feel less negative about himself.

Helping Someone with Borderline Personality Disorder

Have a loved one who's been diagnosed with BPD? While you can't force them to seek treatment, you can take steps to improve communication, set healthy boundaries, and stabilize your relationship.

Learning all you can

If your loved one has borderline personality disorder, it's important to recognize that he or she is suffering. The destructive and hurtful behaviors are a reaction to deep emotional pain. In other words, they're not about you. When your loved one does or says something hurtful towards you, understand that the behavior is motivated by the desire to stop the pain they are experiencing; it's rarely deliberate.

Learning about BPD won't automatically solve your relationship problems, but it will help you understand what you're dealing with and handle difficulties in more constructive ways.

To help someone with BPD, first take care of yourself

When a family member or partner has borderline personality disorder, it's all too easy to get caught up in heroic efforts to please and appease him or her. You may find yourself putting most of your energy into the person with BPD at the expense of your own emotional needs. But this is a recipe for resentment, depression, burnout, and even physical illness. You can't help someone else or enjoy sustainable, satisfying relationships when you're run down and overwhelmed by stress. As in the event of an in-flight emergency, you must "put on your own oxygen mask first."

You're allowed (and encouraged) to have a life!

Give yourself permission to have a life outside of your relationship with the person with BPD. It's not selfish to carve out time for yourself to relax and have fun. In fact, when you return to your BPD relationship, you'll both benefit from your improved perspective.

Learn to manage stress.

Getting anxious or upset in response to problem behavior will only increase your loved one's anger or agitation. By practicing with sensory input, you can learn to relieve stress as it's happening and stay calm and relaxed when the pressure builds.

Avoid the temptation to isolate.

Make it a priority to stay in touch with family and friends who make you feel good. You need the support of people who will listen to you, make you feel cared for, and offer reality checks when needed.

Join a support group for BPD family members.

Meeting with others who understand what you're going through can go a long way. If you can't find an in-person support group in your area, you may want to consider joining an online BPD community.

Don't neglect your physical health.

Eating healthfully, exercising, and getting quality sleep can easily fall by the wayside when you're caught up in relationship drama. Try to avoid this pitfall. When you're healthy and well rested, you're better able to handle stress and control your own emotions and behaviors.

Communication tips with someone who has BPD

It's important to recognize when it's safe to start a conversation. If your loved one is raging, verbally abusive, or making physical threats, now is not the time to talk.

Try to make the person with BPD feel heard.

Don't point out how you feel that they're wrong, try to win the argument, or invalidate their feelings, even when what they're saying is totally irrational.

Talk about things other than the disorder.

You and your loved one's lives aren't solely defined by the disorder, so make the time to explore and discuss other interests. Discussions about light subjects can help to diffuse the conflict between you and may encourage your loved one to discover new interests or resume old hobbies.

Do your best to stay calm, even when the person with BPD is acting out.

Avoid getting defensive in the face of accusations and criticisms, no matter how unfair you feel they are. Defending yourself will only make your loved one angrier. Walk away if you need to give yourself time and space to cool down.

Listen actively and be sympathetic.

Avoid distractions such as the TV, computer, or cell phone. Try not to interrupt or redirect the conversation to your concerns. Set aside your judgment, withhold blame and criticism, and show your interest in what's being said by nodding occasionally or making small verbal comments like "yes" or "uh huh." You don't have to agree with what the person is saying to make it clear that you're listening and sympathetic.

Seek to distract your loved one when emotions rise.

Anything that draws your loved one's attention can work, but distraction is most effective when the activity is also soothing. Try exercising, sipping hot tea, listening to music, grooming a pet, painting, gardening, or completing household chores.

Focus on the emotions, not the words.

The feelings of the person with BPD communicate much more than what the words he or she is using. People with BPD need validation and acknowledgement of the pain they're struggling with. Listen to the emotion your loved one is trying to communicate without getting bogged down in attempting to reconcile the words being used.

Setting healthy boundaries with a borderline loved one

One of the most effective ways to help a loved one with BPD gain control over their behavior is to set and enforce healthy limits or boundaries. Setting limits can help your loved one better handle the demands of the outside world, where schools, work, and the legal system, for example, all set and enforce strict limits on what constitutes acceptable behavior.Establishing boundaries in your relationship can replace the chaos and instability of your current situation with an important sense of structure and provide you with more choices about how to react when confronted by negative behavior. When both parties honor the boundaries, you'll be able to build a sense of trust and respect between you, which are key ingredients for any meaningful relationship.

Setting boundaries is not a magic fix for a relationship, though. In fact, things may initially get worse before they get better. The person with BPD fears rejection and is sensitive to any perceived slight. This means that if you've never set boundaries in your relationship before, your loved one is likely to react badly when you start. If you back down in the face of your loved one's rage or abuse, you'll only be reinforcing their negative behavior and the cycle will continue. But, remaining firm and standing by your decisions can be empowering to you, benefit your loved one, and ultimately transform your relationship.

How to set and reinforce healthy boundaries

Talk to your loved one about boundaries at a time when you're both calm, not in the heat of an argument. Decide what behavior you will and will not tolerate from the person and make those expectations clear.

DO

Make sure everyone in the family agrees on the boundaries and how to enforce the consequences if they're ignored.

Think of setting boundaries as a process rather than a single event. Instead of hitting your loved one with a long list of boundaries all at once, introduce them gradually, one or two at a time.

Calmly reassure the person with BPD when setting limits.

DON'T

- Enable the person with BPD by protecting them from the consequences of their actions. If your loved one won't respect your boundaries and continues to make you feel unsafe, then you may need to leave. It doesn't mean you don't love them, but your self-care should always take priority.

- Make threats and ultimatums that you can't carry out. As is human nature, your loved one will inevitably test the limits you set. If you relent and don't enforce the consequences, your loved one will know the boundary is meaningless and the negative behavior will continue. Ultimatums are a last resort (and again, you must be prepared to follow through).
- Tolerate abusive behavior. No one should have to put up with verbal abuse or physical violence. Just because your loved one's behavior is the result of a personality disorder, it doesn't make the behavior any less real or any less damaging to you or other family members.

Supporting your loved one's BPD treatment

Borderline personality disorder is highly treatable, yet it's common for people with BPD to avoid treatment or deny that they have a problem. Even if this is the case with your loved one, you can still offer support, improve communication, and set boundaries while continuing to encourage your friend or family member to seek professional help. While medication options are limited, the guidance of a qualified therapist can make a huge difference to your loved one's recovery. BPD therapies, such as Dialectical Behavior Therapy (DBT) and schema-focused therapy, can help your loved one work through their relationship and trust issues and explore new coping techniques. In therapy, they can learn how to calm the emotional storm and self-soothe in healthy ways.

How to support treatment

If your loved one won't acknowledge that they have a problem with BPD, you may want to consider couple's therapy. Here, the focus is on the relationship and promoting better communication, rather than on your loved one's disorder. Your partner may more readily agree to this and eventually consider pursuing BPD therapy in the future.

Encourage your loved one to explore healthy ways of handling stress and emotions by practicing mindfulness and employing relaxation techniques such as yoga, deep breathing, or meditation. Sensory-based stimulation can also help them to relieve stress in the moment. Again, you can participate in any of these therapies with your loved one, which can strengthen your bond and may encourage them to pursue other avenues of treatment as well.

By developing an ability to tolerate distress, your loved one can learn how to press pause when the urge to act out or behave impulsively strikes. Help Guide's free Emotional Intelligence Toolkit offers a step-by-step, self-guided program to teach your loved one how to ride the "wild horse" of overwhelming feelings while staying calm and focused.

10 Natural Strategies for People with Borderline Personality Disorder

- Psychotherapy: Many forms of psychotherapy, including cognitive behavioral therapy or dialectical behavioral therapy, may be the first line of defense.
- Family therapy: This can be beneficial to improve relationships with loved ones.
- Brain healthy diet: Eating foods that nourish the brain may be helpful for those struggling with a personality disorder.
- Addressing food sensitivities: Avoiding foods that may increase symptoms can be helpful.
- Foods that are common allergens include sugar, soy, dairy, gluten, corn, artificial dyes, preservatives, and food additives,
- Nutrient supplementation: Vitamin and mineral deficiencies have been associated with a variety of psychiatric conditions. Be sure to get enough of these important nutrients—omega-3 fatty acids, magnesium, vitamin D, and probiotics.

- Eliminating alcohol and drug use.
- Limiting caffeine.
- Exercising daily: Physical activity has mood-boosting benefits.
- Using stress-management techniques to soothe anxiety.

CONCLUSION

- Borderline personality disorder (BPD) is a mental illness that is marked by an ongoing pattern of varying moods, self-image, and behavior.
- Signs/traits of borderline personality disorder include: avoiding abandonment, unstable personal relationships, distorted and unstable self-image, impulsive behaviors, self-harming behavior, periods of intense depressed mood, chronic feelings of boredom or emptiness, inappropriate anger, and cognitive disturbances.
- Underlying causes that can contribute to BPD include: genetics/inheritance, early

traumatic experiences, substance abuse, and abnormal brain function.

- Co-morbidities can make BPD difficult to treat. These include: depression, anxiety, PTSD, eating disorders and substance abuse.

www.ingramcontent.com/pod-product-compliance
Lightning Source LLC
LaVergne TN
LVHW052030170826
845678LV00018B/2487